Take A Fall Retreat At Home

Jennifer Millette

DEDICATION

To all of my students, teachers and friends who have inspired me,
supported me , and retreated with me.

CONTENTS

ACKNOWLEDGMENTS

This book would not have been possible without the encouragement of Anna Castle, Tina Diel, Christine McGrath and Nikki VanderVeen. Thank you for being there when I needed you!   Thank you also to Anna, Tina, and Christine for being my models in the book, and to Anna for offering her studio, Yoga Castle, for our photo shoot.

1 WELCOME TO YOUR FALL RETREAT

"I need to get out of here. I need a retreat!" How many times have you thought that, even said it out loud? Chances are this longing intensifies during rainstorms, bumper to bumper traffic jams or your child's (or boss') meltdown about nothing in particular and everything at once. When life gets crazy, our natural impulse is to lean back and let the world go by, at least for a little while. Whether overwhelmed by external demands or by our own internal expectations not being met, retreats hold that promise and possibility of restoring our settings to neutral.   This is especially true during seasonal transitions. When the seasons change, this is a natural time to regroup, reflect on the season just passed and plan for the season ahead.

I've had the privilege of assisting with several destination yoga and meditation retreats. I've learned lifelong lessons from these experiences at the retreat centers, from my teacher, and from clients themselves. It's especially interesting to notice the changes that occur in the participants over the course of a weeklong retreat. Each person comes with her own set of expectations for the adventure ahead, and usually comes away from the experience with those expectations far surpassed. Coming back from these times away from the 'real world', it's fascinating to observe the changes in those who set their intention to keep up with what they've learned-the self-care, the nurturing choices, the rituals-compared to those who don't. The ones who keep up this lifestyle tend to develop their ability to respond rather to react, to keep their inner glow, manifest more positive changes and experiences in their life, and take any challenges that show up in stride.

My teacher incorporated the ancient art and science of Ayurveda- sister science of yoga-into her retreat teachings. This consciousness-based health care system recognizes and embraces that we are nature and nature is us; we survive and thrive by recognizing its daily and seasonal rhythms, and noting how the natural elements of earth, wind and fire manifest in us

Ayurvedic practices- include yoga and meditation-exist to bring us back into a natural state of balance, of resting ease. One reason that we find retreats so immediately soothing is because they are typically set in beautiful, outside locales. They serve local, fresh seasonal foods for meals, and promote activities that can be done outside in nature. However, these Ayurvedic practices were meant to be utilized in all settings, and can be adapted regardless of weather and location. Another reason that these experiences tend to be so cathartic is that they occur in a state of being truly present, the natural state we instinctively seek out beyond a conscious level.

Based on these observations, I realized a retreat can go beyond a specific place, person or timeframe. It can be an attitude, a lifestyle, a choice to live life from that place, of being perpetually on retreat. Whether you're someone who is not able to physically retreat at this time, or somebody who intuitively senses you need more than a single week or so away to maintain the transformational qualities that such an experience can bring, you can apply and savor these same lessons as well. I invite you to join me in dedicating time to yourself, to welcome these present moment rituals of restoration and renewal into your life, and eventually into your daily routine.

Take a week or so to begin incorporating some of these rituals at home. These practices build upon each other, and their benefits exponentially grow over time. When family and friends notice your innate calm and radiant glow and ask "what have you been doing, simply smile and say "I'm on retreat."

2 RETREAT PRACTICES AND RITUALS

The retreats I have been fortunate enough to be involved with had some or all of these elements to them. Each of them have been specifically chosen to either add nourishment, allow expression, or cleanse toxins from at least one of the koshas (layers) of the self:

Daily Meditation-Meditation allows us to learn to deal with our mind and thoughts, bringing these entities to a place where they work for us instead of struggling against us. Ideally meditation occurs 30 minutes, twice a day, in the morning and late afternoon.

Sit With The Sun-Regardless of outside temperature, observing the sunrise and/or sunset is a humbling, beautiful experience. It reminds us of the beauty of nature and our connection to something greater than ourselves. If you live someplace with minimal exposure to the sun, a seasonal light box works well.

Gratitude Journal- They say happiness is actually a by-product of gratitude. Starting and finishing the day remembering what we're grateful for strengthens our relationships and deepens our connection to the world around us.

Detox Drink- Sip hot water with lemon throughout the day to move and release accumulated toxins (ama), slow ingestion of food sugars, and lower the body's acidity.

Spend Time In Nature-Nature moves on its own timetable, and when we are in it our natural rhythms sync with it. Watching nature unfold in front of us teaches us invaluable life lessons. Do those birds who fly so beautifully together in structured formation have numerous planning meetings and form committees, or do they just know what needs to be done and do it?

Yoga-Yoga unites the body and mind through the breath, clearing any obstructions in the body, mind and heart that prevent us from living our purpose (dharma). It teaches us how to be truly present and comfortable in our bodies, grateful for what they do for us instead of judging them for what we think they lack.

Create Art-Human beings are intuitively creative and have the urge to express this impulse. Choose to let go of old thought patterns (ie, "I'm not good at art") and instead embrace your inner artist. Take time to sketch, paint, collage, make jewelry, cook, take photographs…..anything that inspires you. Creativity takes many forms, just look around and find yours.

Stimulate Digestion-Have ginger tea or fresh ginger steeped in hot water before meals to stimulate digestive fire (agni), preparing the body to receive food and digest it efficiently.

Simple, Delicious Meals-For true nourishment inside and out, choose fresh, local, colorful ingredients to create meals to ensure optimal flavor, health benefits and nutritional value. Food takes on the energy surrounding it, so prepare it from a place of being appreciative for the culinary experience you are about to savor. Meals that require fewer ingredients are satiating without being overwhelming in the preparation phase. A recent favorite of mine is a simple grilled Portobello mushroom, pepper and onion sandwich on toasted tomato focaccia bread, topped with herbed goat cheese. Mouthwatering.

Observe Silence-Our society has come to view silence as something bad or awkward, a situation we must change immediately. Not sure what I mean? Next time you are talking with somebody and a silence comes up, pause a bit rather than rushing to say something, anything to fill it. The stress and anxiety we fill our minds with serves as a similar function, as we rush to fill the silence of our minds. Set time during your day for silence. This can be during the sunrise/sunset, during your commute to or from work, or during a meal where, chances are, you will eat slower, notice the food tastes better, and become fuller while eating less.

Surround Your Senses With Beauty-We are multi-sensory beings and use those senses to take in environmental stimuli. The good news is that have much more control over our surroundings than we may realize. Retreat centers and luxurious spas are deliberately designed to soothe and entice all of our senses from the moment we enter. Make conscious choices to invite beauty in all forms into your settings…..fresh flowers on the table, your favorite aromatherapy oils or spritz close by, music that is pleasing to your ear, soft fabrics, and gorgeous colors are just some ways you can customize your retreat lifestyle.

Nurturing Reading-I freely admit enjoying mindless beach reads and suspenseful crime thrillers, but they don't tap into the power that the written word has for healing. For this purpose, choose inspirational books or literature that engages, rather than numbs the mind, and connects it to your heart. It's often through what we read that new ideas first spark or that we are inspired to finally take positive actions.

3 PLAN YOUR RETREAT

The retreat designed in this book was created specifically to be taken during the fall season. Fall, with its gorgeous colors and crisp smells, is the bridge to the holiday season. It becomes dry, cold, and windy as this transition occurs, and our bodies and minds follow suit.   A fall retreat, therefore, creates warmth to relax and empower you, helping you find quiet and calm during this season of change. The choice of colors, scents, music/sounds, yoga, and menu choices are all very deliberate in that-according to Ayurveda-they are especially useful for this purpose.

CREATE YOUR RETREAT SPACE

It is essential that you have a sacred space during this week for quiet time. Choosing and designing this space for yourself is itself an act of nourishment and creating beauty. Identify a space that you can meditate, journal and practice yoga in that is free from distractions. Then create your space:

- Colors are earthy and pastel, ie khaki, grey, olive, light pinks, yellows and greens.
- Music is calming and relaxing, classical music, slower paced, or nature sounds
- Infuse sweet, warm, relaxing aromatherapy oils or candles like chamomile, geranium, lavender, vanilla, cinnamon, sandalwood
- Select photos, pictures, or other visually rejuvenating art to display
- Alter or small table to display art, sculpture, jewelry, or other meaningful or inspirational personal items
- Meditation cushion
- Yoga mat
- Blanket

PACKING LIST

Going on a retreat involves both physical actions and adjustments in mindsets. Regardless if you are traveling to a destination retreat or taking a retreat at home, you will need to make sure you have the necessary items at your disposal, physically, mentally, emotionally, and situationally.

- Journal
- Nourishing Food and Drink
- Time
- An Open Mind
- Aromatherapy
- Massage Oil-(sesame or almond oil are good choices for fall dry skin)
- Nourishing Reading/Content

YOUR RETREAT ITINERARY

Retreats vary in length, anywhere from 1 day to 1 month. The most common retreat lengths are 3 days (long weekend) or 7 days. Decide what time frame best fits your needs for your fall retreat, look at your schedule, and write it in!

Ideally, we rise with the sun and rest with the sun. This means that we set our daily schedule as close to this as possible, accessing the energy of the dominant energy (called *dosha* in Ayurveda) at its corresponding time of day. Earth (Kapha) times are 6-10am/pm, times of slow transitions to meet the challenges of the day or night ahead. Fire (Pitta) times are 10-2am/pm, times to be productive in terms of activity or sleep. Wind (Vata) times are 2-6 am/pm, times of creativity and developing new ideas.

MORNING: 6-10AM (Slow Transition Time)

- Wake up
- Sit with the sun
- Drink tea or detox drink
- Morning walk (time in nature)

- Yoga
- Meditation
- Gratitude journal
- Breakfast

EARLY AFTERNOON: 10-2PM (Productive Time)

- Complete work
- Eat lunch

LATE AFTERNOON: (Creative Time)

- Have tea or detox drink at 2pm
- Create art or journal
- Meditate again around 5-6pm

EARLY EVENING AND BEDTIME: 6-10PM (Slow Transition Time)

- Eat dinner 6-7pm
- Early bed time, at least 3 hours after dinner
- Minimize reading, eating and watching TV while in bed
- In bed with lights off by 10:30pm

4 MINDFUL MEALS

Food and mealtimes play a starring role in your retreat experience. Anticipation of mealtimes, consuming delicious food, and learning about recipes and healthful benefits of chosen ingredients really support your wellness goals and keep you motivated to stay on track. The opposite is true as well. Think of a beautiful hotel or wonderful vacation you may have taken. If the food is lackluster, it really dims the entire experience. Both menu choices, and decisions around mealtimes and the environment they are presented in, are important to enhance your intentions for your retreat week.

Whether following a focused retreat protocol or simply going about regular day to day life, our choices around food preparation, consumption and elimination are all encompassing. We literally become what we eat! In modern times, however, meal selection is largely based on access, timing and convenience. What can we grab on our thirty minute lunch break? However, with more and more people making the connection to mindless eating and their personal malaise, awareness of alternative eating plans has arisen, often guiding us back to ancient principles for application to modern times. Nutrition viewed from an Ayurvedic perspective looks at food in terms of its taste and energetic properties. We are food and food is us. Potential intentional choices surround every aspect of a meal, from the time of day we eat, from where and with whom its prepared, to where and with whom we consume our food, as well as the décor and sensory accents during and surrounding the meal, the time allotted for the meal itself, and the post-meal experience. All of these factors affect one's ability to completely and cleanly digest the meal.

Ayurveda reminds us to look at nature to see the prana, or life force, shining bright around us. It intuitively follows that the closer we are to nature in our food choices, the more we maintain our intrinsic state of doshic balance that we were born with and destined to maintain. We truly are and become what we eat. Complete digestion is a primary goal and key principle in practicing Ayurveda. We truly are -and therefore become – what we eat. Therefore, to keep ama (the physical, mental and emotional toxins that gradually accumulate within a person over time) low, one needs to jump start their metabolism and stoke their digestive fire by changing what, when and how you eat. At first some of these adjustments may seem a bit foreign or dramatic, but over time these changes can be seamlessly incorporated into your life.

ROUTINES RIGHT FOR YOU

Laura Plumb, author of *Ayurvedic Cooking for Beginners*, simplifies these guidelines into 5 Rights:

Right Quality:

- Prepare or eat homemade foods whenever possible
- Eat freshly prepared foods, no more than 2-3 days stored in refrigerator
- Lightly cooked foods are considered easier to digest, so are generally preferable to raw or overcooked foods
- Increase fruits, vegetables and grains, warm milk or non-dairy milk, nuts and seeds
- Reduce ice-cold beverages since they inhibit digestion

Right Quantity:

- Using a scale of 0-10 (with 0 being starving and 10 being full), start when a 2 or 3, stop when at 6 or 7
- Don't have your next meal when still full from the previous one
- Leave 1/4 to 1/3 of your stomach empty to aid digestion

Right Balance:

- Incorporate the six tastes at every meal, favoring the tastes that serve your intention for the meal/season

Right Timing:

- Use the Ayurvedic clock for meal planning: breakfast and dinner are smaller meals, with your largest meal around noon

Right Mind:

- Prepare foods with love
- Cook with family and friends when possible
- If bringing lunch or dinner to work, make sure you bring something that you actually like, so you are not tempted to go out for local fast food.
- Eat in a quiet, peaceful, comfortable environment
- Eat only when feel hungry
- Do not eat when angry or upset
- Always sit down to eat; when you eat standing your body is in a state of alertness and won't properly begin the digestive process
- Eat at a comfortable pace, chewing slow enough to enjoy the flavor of your food, and completely swallowing each bite before starting the next
- Sit quietly for a few minutes after finishing your meal, noticing the sensations in your body, then take a short walk

THE SIX TASTES

According to Ayurveda, there are six tastes that should be present in every meal: Sweet, Sour, Salty, Pungent, Bitter, Astringent.

Sweet-Sweet is the most grounding and nourishing taste. When eaten in moderation, it promotes longevity, strength, and healthy bodily fluids and tissues. It builds tissues, rejuvenates/nourishes, hydrates, tones muscles, softens/builds skin, hair and voice, boosts longevity, soothes, grounds, strengthens and comforts us, connects, reassures and heals us. Examples of sweet foods include: grains, pasta, rice, bread, starchy vegetables, dairy, meat, chicken, fish, sugar/honey/molasses, most fats, fruits, nuts

Sour-Sour foods stimulate appetite and saliva production, and is balancing in its light, heating, and oily properties. In moderation, the sour taste awakens the thoughts and emotions, and can improve appetite, digestion, and elimination. It cleanses skin, boosts metabolic activity, digestion, firms/strengthens tissues, stimulates sweating, eliminates gas and bloating, improves elimination, increases appetite and salivation, moistens food we eat, creates alertness and sharpness of mind. Examples of sour foods include: citrus fruits, berries, tomatoes, pickled and fermented foods, vinegar, raspberries, tempeh, yogurt

Salty- Salt adds taste to foods, stimulates digestion, helps electrolyte balance, cleanses tissues, and increases absorption of minerals. It boosts digestion, opens blocked channels, improves circulation, softens organs as well as lumps and tumors, decreases general stiffness, increases saliva, is a mild sedative and laxative, awakens mind, strengthens heart, creates a sense of enthusiasm, and builds courage. Examples of salty foods include: sea salt, soy sauce, salted meats, fish, capers, seaweed

Pungent-Pungent food is hot, so stimulates digestion, improves appetite, clears sinuses, stimulates blood circulation, and heightens the senses. It boosts appetite and digestion, opens blocked channels, improves circulation, purifies food, promotes sweating, relieves nerve pain, gives skin a glowing quality, aids in weight loss, helps dissolve fat and toxins, kills parasites, moves blood stagnation. Examples of pungent foods include: spicy peppers/chilies, onions, garlic, cayenne/black pepper, cloves, ginger, mustard, salsa, basil, cardamom, cinnamon, horseradish, oregano, rosemary, thyme, spearmint

Bitter-Bitter is the coolest and lightest of all the tastes. Because of its cool qualities, it's highly physically and mentally detoxifying. -It is a powerful antibacterial, germicidal, antiviral and antiparasitic. It is used to detoxify the body, reduce tissues, purify blood, promote weight loss, create tautness in skin and muscles. It is used as a fat scraper, tonified and cleanser for organs. Examples of bitter foods include: green leafy vegetables, green and yellow vegetables, celery, broccoli sprouts, green tea, mate,

Astringent- Astringent is cool and dry.   Like bitter food, astringent food will help mentally purify and strengthen you. It is an antiseptic, constricts channels that are excessively opened, holds nutrients in body, shrinks pores, controls excess sweating, removes mucus, helps heal sores and wounds, reduces inflammation, cools, slows or stops altogether bleeding as well as diarrhea. Examples of astringent foods include: lentils, dried beans, green apples, grape skins, cauliflower, green beans, asparagus, pomegranates, cranberries, acai berries, teas high in tannins

FALL FOOD GUIDELINES

Ayurvedic teachings help us choose the ideal foods and beverages for a fall time retreat. Fall leaves us prone to dryness, anxiousness and excessive movement, so we balance that with grounding, substantial and filling foods, and increasing sweet, salty, and sour tastes of our meals.

SHOPPING SMARTS
When grocery shopping for your suggested retreat recipes, sure to keep these guidelines in mind:

- Choose unprocessed, whole foods whenever possible
- Choose foods from all colors of the rainbow to ensure getting wide spectrum of vitamins, minerals, nutrients and phytochemicals that are provided by each color group
- Use the Environmental Working Group's Dirty Dozen as a guide to determine which foods have the most pesticides and therefore should be organic. For 2018, they are:
  1. Strawberries
  2. Spinach
  3. Nectarines
  4. Apples
  5. Peaches
  6. Pears

7. Cherries
8. Grapes
9. Celery
10. Tomatoes
11. Sweet Bell Peppers
12. Potatoes

GROCERY LIST

Use the following grocery list as a guide. (If you don't like certain items, feel free to substitute, keeping the fall foods guidelines in mind):

Pantry:

- Oats
- Quinoa
- Basmati rice
- Lentils
- Kidney beans
- Pecans
- Applesauce
- Dried edible lavender (can be found online at Amazon)
- Vegetable broth
- Extra virgin olive oil
- Sesame oil
- Coconut oil

Produce:

Your Choice of Seasonal Fruits: apples, cherries, dates, fresh figs, lemons, raisins

Your Choice of Seasonal Vegetables: carrots, onions, parsnips, shallots, spaghetti squash, red potatoes, cabbage, broccoli, cauliflower, celery, green beans, kale, baby portabella mushrooms, radishes, spinach, zucchini

Dairy:

- Ghee or grass-fed unsalted butter to make your own
- Milk or nut/seed milk of choice

Proteins:

- Eggs
- Smoked Salmon

Spices and Condiments:

- Italian seasoning (or basil and oregano)
- Ground ginger
- Ground cinnamon
- Cloves
- Cardamom
- Cumin
- Garlic
- Nutmeg
- Pepper
- Turmeric
- Sea Salt
- Liquid Aminos

Sweeteners:

- Raw Honey
- Maple Syrup
- Coconut Sugar

5 MENU AND RECIPES

These menu choices are based on a 3 day (long weekend) retreat. If you choose to retreat longer, such as for a week for 10 days, just repeat the meals you liked best or experiment with your own. Use the recipes as templates, feel free to adjust amounts and ingredients to your liking, keeping the fall foods guidelines in mind.

BREAKFAST

- *FALL GRANOLA*
- *OATMEAL*
- *SAVORY BREAKFAST*
- *SALMON AND EGGS*

LUNCH

- *KITCHARI*
- *QUINOA STIR FRY*
- *TRIPLE B SOUP (BEANS, BROCCOLI AND BASMATI RICE)*
- *MINESTRONE*

DINNER

- *PORTABELLA MUSHROOM BISQUE*
- *ITALIAN LENTIL AND KALE SOUP*
- *ROASTED CAULIFLOWER AND CARROTS MEDLEY*
- *SPAGHETTI SQUASH MARINARA*

BEVERAGES

- *FALL DIGESTIVE TEA*
- *FALL CHAI TEA*
- *APPLE CIDER LATTE*
- *LAVENDER HERBAL LATTE*

FALL GRANOLA

Ingredients:

- 2 cups rolled oats
- 1/4 cup water
- 2 tablespoons maple syrup
- 2 tablespoons ground flaxseeds
- 1 tablespoon coconut oil
- 1 teaspoon cinnamon
- 1/2 teaspoon ground cardamom
- 1/4 cup chopped pecans
- 1/4 cup chopped figs

Directions:

- Preheat the oven to 375ºF.
- Coat a large baking sheet (with sides) with coconut oil.
- Stir oats, water, maple syrup, flaxseeds, oil, cinnamon, and cardamom in a large bowl. Stir well to combine.
- Spread mixture on baking sheet and bake for 20 minutes, stirring carefully once or twice.
- Add the pecans and figs and bake an additional 5 minutes.
- Remove and cool completely before storing in an airtight container at room temperature for up to 1 week.

OATMEAL

Ingredients:

- Oatmeal (rolled or steel cut oats)
- Water or milk of choice (to cook with oatmeal)
- Applesauce
- Dates, raisins figs
- Cinnamon

Directions:

- Prepare oatmeal according to directions.
- Heat dates, raisins, and or figs (in separate pan) over medium heat with enough water to cover bottom of pan.
- Once fruit is cooked tender, stir in applesauce and sprinkle of cinnamon.
- Heat fruit and applesauce through, about 1-2 minutes.
- Add fruit mixture to oatmeal in pan and stir.
- Spoon into bowls, top with sprinkle of cinnamon and serve.

SAVORY BREAKFAST

Ingredients:

- 2 red or sweet Potatoes
- ½ cup cabbage
- 1 tbsp olive oil
- Sea salt to taste
- Liquid aminos (optional)

Directions:

- Chop up potatoes and cabbage.
- add in olive oil and massage it in to the potatoes and cabbage.
- Add sea salt, a bit of liquid aminos (optional), and whatever else you'd like.
- Bake at 400 for 20-30 minutes, stir at about 20 minutes.
- Spoon into bowls and serve.

SALMON AND EGGS

Ingredients:

- 2 eggs
- 1 tbsp olive oil, ghee, or other cooking oil
- Smoked salmon
- Capers (optional)

Directions:

- Whisk eggs in bowl.
- Heat pan with oil to cook eggs.
- Pour eggs in pan, continuously stir as they firm.
- Remove cooked eggs from heat.
- Place smoked salmon on plate, add eggs next to or on top, optional topping with capers. Serve.

KITCHARI

Ingredients:

- ½ cup cooked organic white basmati rice
- ¼ cup cooked lentils or split yellow mung beans
- 1-2 cups water
- 2-3 tsp ghee or olive oil
- ¼ tsp coriander
- ¼ tsp cumin
- 1/8-1/4 tsp red chili or cayenne pepper
- ¼ tsp ground ginger
- ¼ tsp turmeric
- Sea salt to taste
- 2 c chopped vegetables like zucchini, chard, leeks
- ½ c spinach leaves, washed and finely chopped
- 1 tsp lemon juice

Directions:

- Heat ghee or oil in pot on medium heat, then add coriander, cumin, turmeric, red chili, and ginger; sauté for 1-2 minutes.
- Add chopped vegetables, toss in oil to coat, sauté for 5-10 minutes (add a bit of water if necessary).
- Add the mung lentils, basmati rice, vegetables, remaining water, and salt; bring to a boil then turn heat to low.
- Cook for 10-15 minutes. Top with spinach and fresh lemon juice.
- Spoon into bowls and serve.

Option: to make this more of a soup, simply add more water and seasonings to taste.

QUINOA STIR FRY

Ingredients:

- 1 tsp minced garlic
- 1 tsp minced onion
- 1 tbsp Sesame oil
- ½ cup diced carrots
- ½ cup halved green beans
- ½ cup chopped broccoli
- ½ chopped cauliflower
- ½ cup Cooked quinoa
- Sea Salt to taste
- ½ tsp garlic powder
- 1 tsp cumin
- ½ tsp coriander
- ½ tsp turmeric

Directions:

- Add minced garlic and onion to heated sesame oil.
- Add carrots, green beans, broccoli and cauliflower and sauté.
- Add cooked quinoa about halfway through cooking veggies.
- Add spices to taste.
- Stir to coat, heat over med heat for 10 minutes.
- Spoon into bowls and serve

(TRIPLE B SOUP (BEANS, BROCCOLI AND BASMATI RICE)

Ingredients:

- 1 tsp fresh minced garlic
- 1 tsp dried minced onion
- 1 tbsp olive oil
- 1 tbsp miso
- 1 tsp italian seasoning
- ½ cup broccoli
- ½ cup cooked kidney beans
- ½ cup cooked basmati rice,
- 1 tbsp nutritional yeast
- 1 tbsp liquid aminos
- Sea salt to taste
- 1 tsp garlic powder
- 4 cups water

Directions:

- Heat oil to medium heat and sauté minced garlic and onion.
- Add broccoli and sauté until al dente.
- Add kidney beans, and water to cover.
- Add nutritional yeast, liquid aminos, salt, garlic powder, Italian seasoning and miso.
- Stir and adjust spices and water to taste. Make sure there is enough water that it is a soup instead of a stir fry.
- Let simmer over medium-low heat for 10-20 minutes.
- Spoon into bowls and serve.

MINESTRONE SOUP

Ingredients:

- 4 cups water
- ½ cup cooked Basmati Rice or pasta of choice
- ½ cup cooked Pinto and/or kidney beans
- ½ cup diced carrots
- ½ cup kale or spinach
- ½ cup diced celery
- 1 tbsp olive oil
- ½ tsp garlic powder
- ½ cup onions
- ½ tsp cumin
- ½ tsp turmeric
- ¼ tsp black pepper
- ¼ tsp coriander
- ½ tsp basil
- ½ oregano
- Sea salt to taste

Directions:

- Sauté garlic and onions in oil.
- Add carrots, celery, kale to oil (to cover bottom of pan), continue to sauté.
- Add spices to sautéed veggies, cover with water.
- Add rice/pasta, beans, and more water to pot, seasoning to taste. Aim for 2-3 times as much liquid as veggies, rice and beans.
- Bring to brief boil, lower to med-low heat, simmer for 10-20 minutes or to taste.
- Spoon into bowls and serve.

PORTABELLA MUSHROOM BISQUE

Ingredients:

- ½ cup baby portabellas
- ½ cup onions
- 1 tbsp liquid aminos
- Sea salt to taste
- 1 tbsp coconut oil
- 3 cups vegetable broth or water
- 1 cup milk of choice (if non dairy, make sure it's plain and unsweetened)

Directions:

- Sauté above ingredients with a bit of veggie broth over medium heat.
- Pour sautéed mixture into Vitamix and add more broth to cover (about 2-3 times as much broth as veggies).
- Puree and return mixture to pot over medium heat.
- Add milk, more broth and liquid aminos to taste.
- Spoon into bowls and serve.

For chunkier mushroom bisque, reserve 1-2 handfuls of chopped baby portabellas after they are sautéed

ITALIAN LENTIL AND KALE SOUP

Ingredients:

- 1 tsp minced garlic
- 1 tsp minced onion
- 1 tbsp olive oil
- ½ cup diced celery
- ½ cup ripped kale
- 1 tsp Italian seasoning blend
- Sea salt to taste
- ½ tsp garlic powder
- ½ tsp celery seed
- 1 tsp liquid aminos
- ½ cup cooked lentils
- 4 cups of water

Directions

- sauté garlic and oil in oil.
- add celery to simmer 1 minute or so, then add splash of water.
- add half cup of water and kale, stir to coat, leave over medium heat 3-5 minutes.
- add all spices, squeeze or splash of liquid aminos, stir to coa.t
- add 8 cups water, stir and bring to boil before reducing heat to medium. Taste and adjust spices, salt and liquid aminos.
- Add cooked lentils, make sure can see liquid through the lentils (ratio), heat at medium for 10 minutes.
- Pulse with immersion blender to desired consistency, cook for another 10-20 minutes over medium heat.
- Spoon into bowls and serve.

ROASTED CAULIFLOWER AND CARROTS MEDLEY

Ingredients:

- 1 cup chopped cauliflower
- 1 cup carrot chunks
- 1 tbsp olive oil
- ½ tsp garlic powder
- ½ tsp cumin
- ½ tsp coriander
- ½ tsp turmeric
- Sea salt to taste

Directions:

- Preheat oven to 400 degrees
- Toss cauliflower and carrots in oil and spices
- Roast vegetable on oil coated pan approximately 20 minutes, turn vegetables about halfway through cooking
- Spoon into bowls and serve

SPAGHETTI SQUASH MARINARA

Ingredients:

- 1 Spaghetti squash
- 1 tbsp olive oil
- 1 tsp minced garlic
- Marinara sauce (can be organic store bought or your favorite recipe)

Directions:

- Preheat oven to 400 degrees
- Place squash in oven and roast for approximately 40 minutes
- Take squash out of oven and let cool to the touch (approximately 30 minutes)
- Slice squash in half and scrape out 'spaghetti' strands. Reserve seeds for roasting later on if you choose
- Add squash spaghetti to pan with heated olive oil and sautéed garlic. Stir to coat, approximately 2-3 minutes
- Add marinara sauce to pan, stir to coat and warm through
- Spoon into bowls and serve

SAVORY SPICE MIX

Spices are a key component of Ayurvedic cooking, due to the ability they have to balance our bodies and minds. Use this mix as you would any general seasoning mix.

Ingredients:

- 2 tbsp cumin
- 2 tbsp coriander
- 1 tbsp turmeric
- 1 tbsp ground ginger
- ½ tsp cardamom
- ¼ tsp sea salt

Directions:

- Combine ingredients in airtight jar, store and use when preparing dishes that call for spices or flavoring.

GHEE (CLARIFIED BUTTER)

Ghee is one of the most important foods in Ayurvedic cooking. Cooking off the casein proteins and fat cells are cooked off to produce a healthy fat that supports immunity, rejuvenation and digestion.

Ingredients:

- 1 lb pure unsalted grass fed butter (preferably organic)

Directions:

- Melt butter in a medium sauce pan over medium heat; bring to boil then reduce heat to medium low.
- The ghee will foam and gurgle as it releases steam; once it gets quiet reduce heat to low.
- Carefully (don't stir the butter) separate foam from top of the butter; if butter is transparent to the bottom the ghee is done-otherwise cook another minute or two.
- Strain ghee through fine mesh strainer with cheesecloth into a clean glass jar
- Let ghee cool, then store unrefrigerated, tightly sealed glass jar. It keeps indefinitely.

FALL DIGESTIVE TEA

Ingredients:

- 1 cup water per serving
- 1/8 tsp ground ginger per serving
- ¼ tsp lemon juice per serving

Directions:

- Heat water to just under boiling, pour into mug.
- Add ginger and lemon juice.
- Stir and serve

FALL CHAI TEA

Ingredients:

- 3 cups filtered water
- 1 tsp ground cardamom
- ½ tsp cloves
- 1 cinnamon sticks or 1 tsp ground cinnamon
- ¼ tsp ground ginger (add more to taste)
- 1 cup preferred milk
- *Optional: Coconut sugar or honey*

Directions:

- Combine above ingredients except sugar in saucepan.
- boil then reduce to medium heat for 5 minutes.
- Take off heat and let steep for 5 more minutes.
- Strain into mugs, add coconut sugar if you like, and serve.

APPLE CIDER LATTE

Ingredients:

- ¾ cup apple cider
- ¼ cup milk of choice
- ¼ tsp cinnamon
- 1 tsp maple syrup

Directions:

- Heat apple cider and milk in pan (can adjust ratio to taste) over medium heat.
- Once heated, stir in cinnamon and maple syrup.
- Pour into mug and serve.

LAVENDER HERBAL LATTE

Ingredients:

- ¼ tsp dried edible lavender buds per cup
- ½ cup water
- ½ cup milk of choice
- 1 tsp maple syrup

Directions:

- Heat dried lavender and water milk in pan (can adjust ratio to taste) over medium heat. Let heat for 5 minutes, then add milk.
- Once heated through, strain and pour into mug.
- Stir in maple syrup and serve.

6 RESTFUL SLEEP

A key component of any successful retreat is plenty of time for rest, relaxation, and more rest! Restful sleep is essential for health and longevity. The hours between 10pm and 12 midnight are the most important hours for sleep, as this is when the body and mind digest the day, and make necessary repairs.

Set your goal to be in bed with the lights out by 10:30pm to get the best rest possible. The majority of people in this day and age aren't used to going to bed this early and may consider this an impossible task, but it can be done and you will feel significantly better the next day, with more energy, focus and productivity in your work. For a gradual transition to this healthier bedtime, shift all parts of your bedtime routine earlier by half an hour each week until you are in bed by 10:30pm or the desired time. In addition to regulating the bedtime schedule, utilize the following tips to establish a nourishing, peaceful routine to help you fall-and stay-asleep:

- If you like taking baths, run a hot bath about an hour or so before bed, using aromatherapy essential oil such as lavender, sandalwood or vanilla, soft lights and relaxing music.
- After your bath, have a cup of hot tea or warm milk
- If your mind is very active, journal for a few minutes before bed. This downloads those perseverative or repeating thoughts so you don't keep replaying them when you shut your eyes.
- Make a short to-do list for the next day, to prevent those nagging thoughts that might keep you up ("I have to remember to…."). Knowing they're on the list takes them off of your brain for the time being.
- Read a few minutes worth of inspirational or spiritual literature. Books with short chapters, or magazines with brief articles work well. Make sure this is an actual paper book, however, not a kindle or iPad, as the light can disrupt natural rhythms. (see next two suggestions)

- Refrain from watching television, working, or otherwise using your computer or phone while you are in bed. This keeps you focused on the outside world and not on preparing yourself to rest.
- All electronics should be turned off at least one hour before bedtime, to allow time to unplug and retreat and minimize the effects of their blue light, which too close to bedtime has been found to interfere with sleep.
- Once in bed, close your eyes and simply feel your body. Start from the crown of the head and go all the way to the tips of the toes, scanning for any areas of tightness that you can breathe softness into. If you notice tension in specific parts of the body, briefly contract (tense) the muscles, then relax them.
- If you have trouble falling asleep, listen to a guided visualization or yoga nidra script, just noticing the natural ebb and flow of your breath until you fall asleep.

7 MEDITATION PRACTICE

MUDRAS

Mudras are often used during meditation practice. Mudras have been called yoga poses for the hands. They are hand positions with specific intentions behind them, that have been said to promote specific effects/experiences within a person. You can use them during meditation, or anytime you feel the need.

Wisdom Mudra (Gyan Mudra)

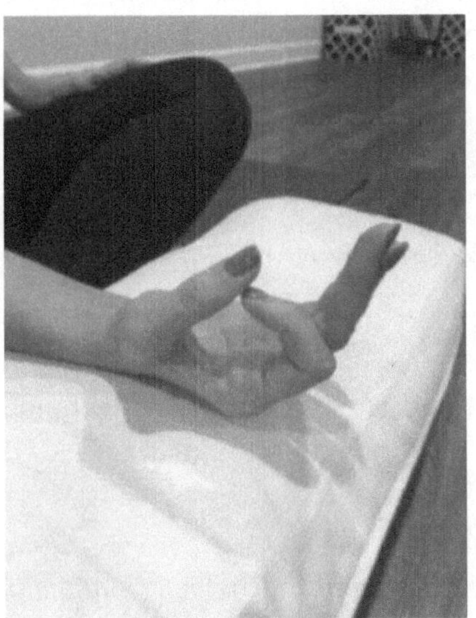

Cueing:

Make the 'ok' sign with each hand, tips of index fingers and thumbs to touch. Slide tip of index finger nail onto the pad of each thumb. Rest hands on thighs or let arms rest next to sides.

Benefits:

- Alleviates anxiety
- Quiets the mind
- Increases lung capacity

MEDITATION

Mindful Breath Meditation

Breath observance is one of the most common mindfulness techniques. The focus stays on an entire breath, from beginning to end. This just means purely observing the breath as it is, without changing it in any way. When you are focused on what is happening in the moment, your mind is unable to ruminate on the past, or worry about the future. The result is your natural, resting state of peace.

Cueing: Take a comfortable seat, using any props you need for comfort. As you inhale, think "Inhaling in". As you exhale, think "Exhaling out". Continue thinking "Inhaling in" on your inhale, and "Exhaling out" on your exhale. Your mind might start to slow a bit, this is ok. If your thoughts start to wander to other topics, just gently guide your mind back to your breath, silently repeating "Inhaling in…..Exhaling out….". Meditate for about 5-30 minutes.

RELAXING BREATHWORK (PRANAYAMA)

Belly Breath

Due to the mindful aspects of this breathing technique, it could also be used in place of or in addition to Mindful Breath Meditation.

Cueing:

Sitting up tall, place both hands at the belly. Inhale and feel belly filling up with space from the breath. Exhale and feel the belly emptying the space from the breath. Can also be done reclined, at the beginning or end of yoga practice, or before bedtime.

Benefits:

- Calms the body
- Soothes the mind
- Settles strong emotions
- Oxygenates the tissues

8 YOGA PRACTICE

The following yoga practice and poses help relax, ground and empower. Intentions for practice include stabilizing, empowering, and releasing excess energy. An affirmation that supports these practices is "There is an earth below me and a universe that supports me." You can take time during any of the poses to breathe and silently repeat this affirmation.

RELAXING YOGA SEQUENCE:

Hold poses for approximately 1-3 minutes, as long as you are comfortable, except for Relaxation, which can be held for 5-15 minutes. Make sure to take asymmetrical poses to both sides

- *Child's Pose (Bal asana)*
- *Low Lunge (Anjaney asana)*
- *Warrior I (Virabhadr asana I)*
- *Warrior II (Virabhadr asana II)*
- *Tree (Vrks asana))*
- *Standing Forward Fold (Uttan asana)*
- *Bound Angle (Baddhakon asana)*
- *Reclined Spinal Twist (Supta Matsyendr asana)*
- *Corpse or Relaxation Pose (Shav asana or Sav asana)*

Child's Pose (Bal asana)

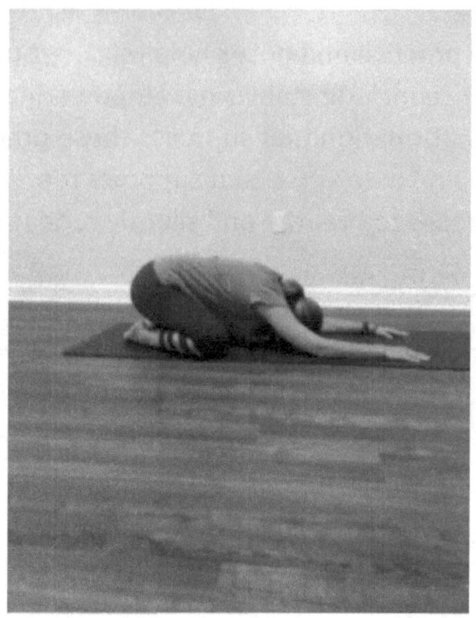

Cueing:

Start in Table

Exhale, draw sitz bones toward heels. Externally rotate thighs so big toes touch
Exhale, flex torso onto mat, rest head on mat or block.

Benefits:

- Relieves stress
- Serves as a resting pose
- Stretches the thighs, hips, ankles and knee

Low Lunge (Anjaney asana)

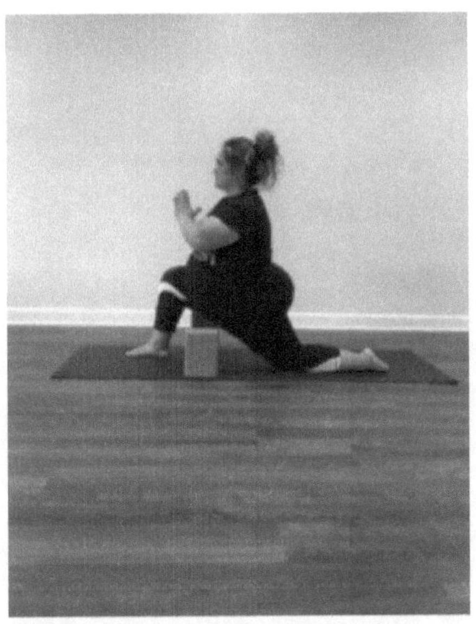

Cueing:

Start with hands and knees on mat.

Inhale, big step forward with right foot between hands. Place hands at hips or reach arms overhead shoulder distance apart.
Exhale, flex front knee in line with ankle.
Inhale, lift up through heart center.
Exhale, square hips to front of mat.

Benefits:

- Anchors a spinning mind
- Alleviates anxiety
- Helps develop balance and coordination
- Encourages focus and communication
- Lengthens and strengthens the arms, shoulders and back

Warrior I (Virabhadr asana I)

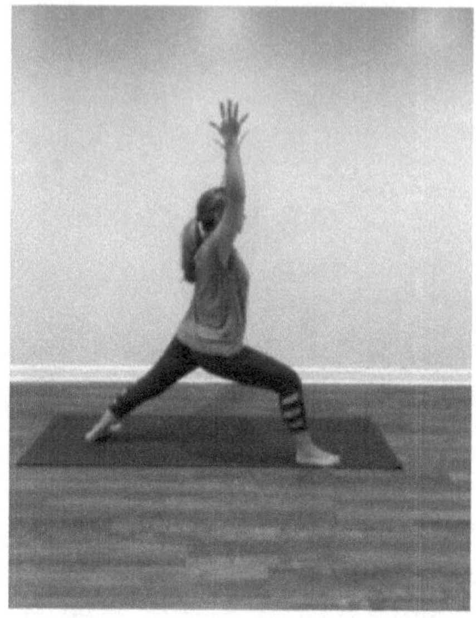

Cueing:

Start standing at front of mat.

Inhale, big step back with left foot, reach arms overhead shoulder distance apart. Externally rotate back hip so outer edge of back foot presses into mat.
Exhale, flex front knee in line with ankle.
Inhale, extend through spine, lift up through heart center.
Exhale, square hips to front of mat.

Benefits:

- Anchors a spinning mind
- Alleviates anxiety
- Helps develop balance and coordination
- Encourages focus and communication
- Lengthens and strengthens the arms, shoulders and back

Warrior II (Virabhadr asana II)

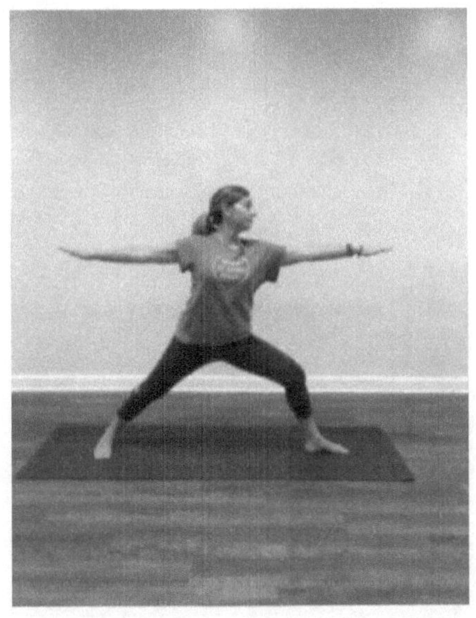

Cueing:

Start standing at front of mat.

Inhale, big step back with right foot, reach right arm straight back and left arm straight forward. Externally rotate back hip so outer edge of back foot presses into mat.
Exhale, flex front knee in line with ankle.
Inhale, extend through spine, lift up through heart center.
Exhale, deepen external rotation of right hip.

Benefits:

- Anchors a spinning mind
- Alleviates anxiety
- Helps develop balance and coordination
- Encourages focus and communication
- Lengthens and strengthens the arms, shoulders and back

Tree (Vrks asana)

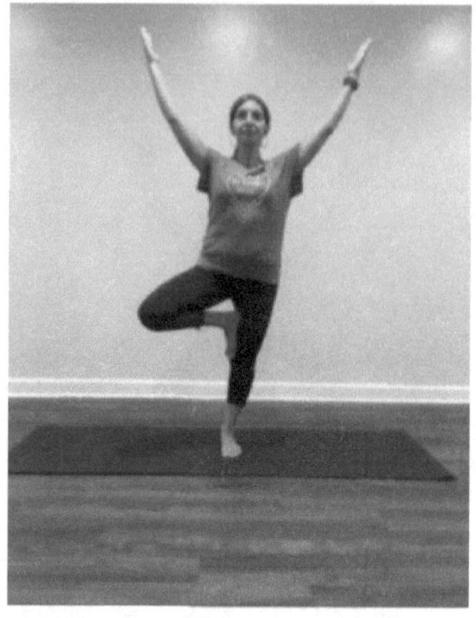

Cueing:

Start standing at front of mat.

Inhale, float right heel off mat and flex right knee.
Exhale, externally rotate right hip, draw right heel above left ankle.
Hold position or slide sole of right foot along inside of left leg, mindful to not actively push on the left knee.
Inhale take hands to heart or reach arms up toward sky.

Benefits:

- Opens the hips
- Lengthens the thigh muscles
- Improves posture and core strength

Standing Forward Fold (Uttan asana)

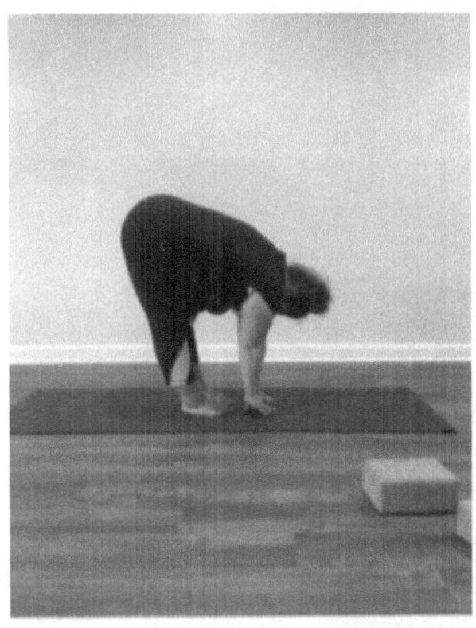

Cueing:

Start standing at front of mat.

Inhale, reach arms up toward sky.
Exhale, flex from hips so hands touch the ground or shins.

Benefits:

- Calms nervous system
- Rejuvenates and relieves fatigue
- Stretches the whole back side of the body, neck to heels
- Helps improve concentration
- Stimulates internal organ function, improves digestive function

Bound Angle Pose (Baddha Kon asana)

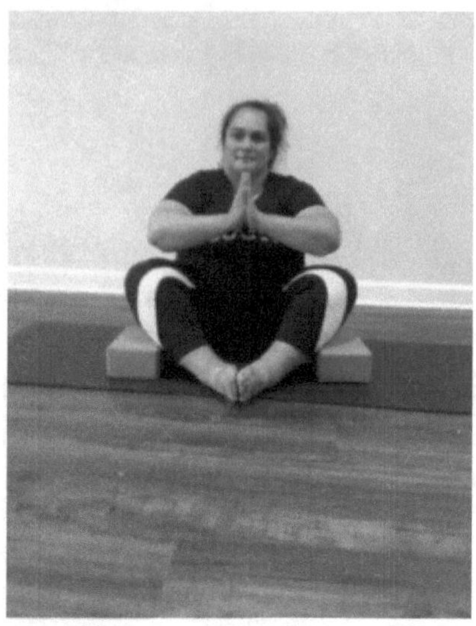

Cueing:

Start seated with legs straight in front of you.

Inhale, flex both knees.
Exhale, externally rotate both hips and draw feet close in towards sitz bones. Press outer edges of the feet together and place thumbs on ball mounts of big toes.

Benefits:

- Stimulates abdominal organs
- Stimulates the heart and improves general circulation
- Stretches the inner thighs, groins, and knees
- Helps relieve mild depression, anxiety, and fatigue
- Soothes menstrual discomfort and sciatica

Reclined Spinal Twist (Supta Matsyendr asana)

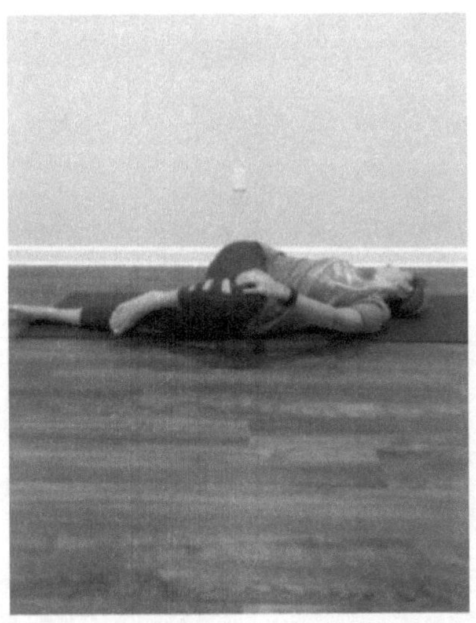

Cueing:

Start Supine (reclined on back)

Exhale, flex right knee into chest.
Inhale, extend spine, placing left hand on right thigh and extending right arm out to right side.
Exhale, cross right knee over to left side, resting right leg on the ground or a prop.

Benefits:

- Strengthens core and side waist muscles
- Enhances brain functioning
- Lengthens postural muscles of the spine
- Tones kidneys to improve digestive function
- Releases toxins

Corpse or Relaxation Pose (Shav asana or Sav asana)

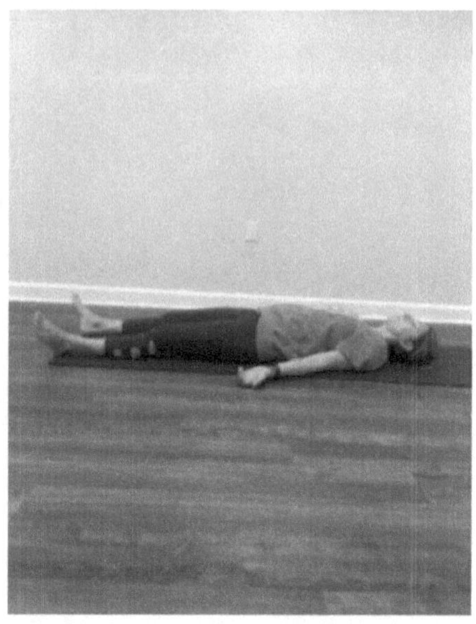

Cueing:

Start in Supine (reclined on back).

Inhale, extend through spine, lift up through heart center and widen collarbones.
Exhale, externally rotate hips and shoulders so feet face corners of mat and palms face up. Allow arms and legs to rest extended on mat.

Benefits:

- Allows the muscles to release tightness, tension and toxins
- Quiets the mind
- Lengthens the spine
- Allows the shoulders and neck to relax

9 RETREAT FOR LIFE

Now that you know how to bring these self-care practices into your home, whenever you need them, your eyes are now opened to new possibilities. Your retreat tools can be used anytime you want or need them. You will be more empowered, more mindful and more compassionate towards yourself and others. Best of luck to you on this new journey of health, happiness and healing.

REFERENCES

BOOKS

Chopra, Deepak, MD. *Perfect Health.* New York, NY: Three Rivers Press; 1991, R 2000.

Davidji. *Secrets of Meditation.* Carlsbad, CA: Hay House Inc; 2012

Jenson, Bernard, PhD, The Chemistry of Man. Warsaw, IN: Whitman Publications; 1983

Kabat-Zinn J, University of Massachusetts Medical C. *Full Catastrophe Living : Using the Wisdom of Your Body and Mind to Face Stress, Pain, and Illness.* New York, N.Y.: Delta Trade Paperbacks; 2005.

Kshirsagar, Suhas, MD. *The Hot Belly* Diet. New York, NY: Atria Books; 2014

Lad, Vasant, MD. *Ayurveda: The Science of Self-Healing.* Santa Fe, NM: Lotus Press; 1984.

Plumb, Laura. *Ayurvedic Cooking for Beginners.* Emeryville, CA: Rockridge Press; 2018

Rosenthal, Joshua. *Integrative Nutrition.* New York, NY: Integrative Nutrition Publishing; 2017

Satchinanada, Sri Swami. *The Yoga Sutras of Patanjali.* Ashland, OH: Integral Yoga Publications; 2012

Silcox, Katie. *Healthy Happy Sexy: Ayurveda Wisdom for Modern Women.* Hillsboro, OR: Beyond Words; 2015.

Yarema, Thomas MD et al. *Eat Taste Heal: An Ayurvedic Guidebook and Cookbook for Modern Living.* Kapaa, HI: Five Elements Press; 2010

WEBSITES

https://www.ewg.org/foodnews/dirty-dozen.php

www.yogajournal.com/poses

FREE GUIDED MEDITATION SCRIPTS AND DOWNLOADS

http://www.chopra.com/articles/guided-meditations

http://www.innerhealthstudio.com/meditation-scripts.html

PROGRAMS OFFERING PERSONAL MANTRAS

Chopra Center-Primordial Sound Meditation (PSM)

http://www.chopra.com/online-courses/primordial-sound-meditation/on-demand#sm.000011af3bkgbdfkaw6j53wcpiqs6

Maharishi Mahesh-Transcendental Meditation (TM)

http://www.tm.org/

ABOUT THE AUTHOR

I am a yoga and meditation teacher, licensed massage therapist, Reiki
Master, and Ayurvedic Health Coach. My specialties include stress
relief, relaxation, energy work, weight loss and behavioral change. I've
always been fascinated how the wisdom of nature, if we choose to
follow it, always guides us toward happiness and health. I also believe
sustainable wellness involves addressing all aspects of the individual. I
have personally experienced the toll that stress and anxiety can take on
the body and mind, and have successfully used the tools I share with
clients in my own life. My work emphasizes alignment of all aspects of
the self; physical, energetic, mental, emotional and spiritual. I I draw
upon the wisdom of Ayurveda, the chakra energy system, and the
recent field of positive psychology so clients can effortlessly incorporate
these strategies into everyday life. I am also a certified trainer through
the National Academy of Sports Medicine, as well as an Approved CE
Provider for Yoga Alliance and NCBTMB for Ayurveda, yoga, meditation
and Reiki. I live, work and play in Frankfort, a southern suburb of
Chicago.